Depression

A Quick Guild To
Meaning & Management
Tips

By:

La Jon Dantzler

TABLE OF CONTENTS

INTRODUCTION..3

What is depression? 5

Types of depression 6

Causes 8

Symptoms 10

Who gets depressed?..14

Depression Treatment Options 23

Depression Tips to Handle the Condition 28

CONCLUSION 31

INTRODUCTION

A very common habit among youngsters is to use the line, "I am depressed!", when they are simply sad or upset. People don't realise the enormity of the word depression and tend to use it as a substitute to sadness.

Most often we think that depression is just a case of extreme sadness. When we are faced with a tragedy, we feel depressed. But after a while it goes away. That's what the general belief is. But depression is far more than a mere bout of sadness. It is something with the potential to cause extreme harm and ruin lives if not treated appropriately.

Keeping the magnitude in mind, let me shine some light on what exactly depression entails.

Depression is a state of being where a person tends to feel absolutely empty, anxious and lost. It is the lowest point on the emotional scale and is marked by a variety of negative feelings like, guilt, helplessness, anger, irritability, etc.

Depression is much more than an extreme mood swing. It is a behavioural disorder, which like any disorder needs treatment. No matter how happy a person may be, if there is depression, it needs to be treated.

People with depression appear to have physical changes in their brains. The significance of these changes is still uncertain, but may eventually help pinpoint causes.

Brain chemistry

Neurotransmitters are naturally occurring brain chemicals that likely play a role in depression. Recent research indicates that changes in the function and effect of these neurotransmitters and how they interact with neurocircuits involved in maintaining mood stability may play a significant role in depression and its treatment.

Hormones

Changes in the body's balance of hormones may be involved in causing or triggering depression. Hormone changes can result with pregnancy and during the weeks or months after delivery (postpartum) and from thyroid problems, menopause or a number of other conditions.

Inherited traits

Depression is more common in people whose blood relatives also have this condition. Researchers are trying to find genes that may be involved in causing depression.

SYMPTOMS

Although depression may occur only once during your life, people typically have multiple episodes. During these episodes, symptoms occur most of the day, nearly every day and may include:

Self-loathing

Strong feelings of worthlessness or guilt. You harshly criticize yourself for perceived faults and mistakes.

Reckless behavior.

You engage in escapist behavior such as substance abuse, compulsive gambling, reckless driving, or dangerous sports.

Concentration problems.

Trouble focusing, making decisions, or remembering things.

Feelings of helplessness and hopelessness.

A bleak outlook—nothing will ever get better and there's nothing you can do to improve your situation.

Loss of interest in daily activities.

You don't care anymore about former hobbies, past times, social activites, or sex. You've lost your ability to feel joy & pleasure.

Appetite or weight changes.

Significant weight loss or weight gain—a change of more than 5% of body weight in a month.

Sleep changes.

Either insomnia, especially waking in the early hours of the morning, or oversleeping.

Anger or irritability.

Feeling agitated, restless, or even violent. Your tolerance level is low, your temper short, and everything and everyone gets on your nerves.

Loss of energy.

Feeling fatigued, sluggish, and physically drained. Your whole body may feel heavy, and even small tasks are exhausting or take longer to complete.

For many people with depression, symptoms usually are severe enough to cause noticeable problems in day-to-day activities, such as work, school, social activities or relationships with others. Some people may feel generally miserable or unhappy without really knowing why.

Depression symptoms in children and teens

Depression Symptoms In Older Adults

Depression is not a normal part of growing older, and it should never be taken lightly. Unfortunately, depression often goes undiagnosed and untreated in older adults, and they may feel reluctant to seek help. Symptoms of depression may be different or less obvious in older adults, such as:

- Memory difficulties or personality changes
- Physical aches or pain
- Fatigue, loss of appetite, sleep problems or loss of interest in sex — not caused by a medical condition or medication
- Often wanting to stay at home, rather than going out to socialize or doing new things
- Suicidal thinking or feelings, especially in older men.

Common signs and symptoms of depression in children and teenagers are similar to those of adults, but there can be some differences.

- In younger children, symptoms of depression may include sadness, irritability, clinginess, worry, aches and pains, refusing to go to school, or being underweight.

- In teens, symptoms may include sadness, irritability, feeling negative and worthless, anger, poor performance or poor attendance at school, feeling misunderstood and extremely sensitive, using recreational drugs or alcohol, eating or sleeping too much, self-harm, loss of interest in normal activities, and avoidance of social interaction.

WHO GETS DEPRESSED?

Depression is common, affecting about 121 million people worldwide. In the United States, it's estimated that in any given year depressive disorders are estimated to affect approximately 18.8 million American adults, or about 9.5% of the U.S. population age 18 and older.

In terms of gender, depression affects both sexes. Unfortunately, depression has had a reputation of being a women's condition, but this is incorrect. Actually more than 6 million men in the U.S. have depression each year.

The symptoms of depression in men are similar to the symptoms of depression in women. But men tend to express those symptoms differently.

How do men and women express depression differently?

In women, depression may be more likely to cause feelings of sadness and worthlessness. Depression in men, on the other hand, may be more likely to cause them to be irritable, aggressive, or hostile.

Either way, the depressed person is suffering, and those around them suffer as well. Therefore, adopting an immediate, problem-solving attitude is essential. Everyone - the depressed person, family, friends, co-workers - benefits by this 'let's get this resolved' approach. Be sure to check out every one of these physically-generated causes of depression:

Toxic metals.

Modern people are exposed to toxic metals from the dental substances in their mouths, from drinking water, food, air and more. A toxic metal body burden can produce very deep-seated and profound depression - absolute hopelessness and despair.

This is also true during a metals detoxification process, which is why it's always essential to undertake even the diagnosis of toxic metals under the guidance of a skilled and experienced professional. The good news is that the depression flushes right out with the metals.

Toxic chemicals.

These are everywhere now in the modern world. Estimates say that each individual is exposed to some 100,000 with more added daily.

A quiet study was conducted in which surgeons were asked to remove a small piece of fat from each patient while conducting the operation. These were then sent into a central laboratory and tested for chemicals. The fat sample with the lowest number listed well over 200 toxic chemicals! For some reason the results of this study never made the headlines.

Many of these cause depression by mimicking sex hormones, where they get into the cell receptors the body's own sex hormones should be regulating.

Just as with toxic chemicals, the services of a competent and skilled practitioner are required to detox these chemicals safely and effectively, and again, any depressive symptoms they cause disappear right along with the chemicals.

Low Thyroid (T1 Or T4):

Revealed by a blood test or muscle testing, this symptom can often turn around by increasing dietary intake or even supplementing with iodine along with removing all sources of exposure to fluoride, including fluoridated drinking water, toothpaste and dental sealants. Fluoride knocks iodine out of the thyroid, causing low thyroid functioning and thus leads directly to depression.

Low Blood Sugar.

This condition causes depression in a manner similar to that of anemia, only in this instance the problem is not getting enough oxygen to the brain, but getting enough blood sugar to the brain. Physical problems such as diabetes, syndrome X (also called metabolic syndrome) can produce this symptom if not properly managed. Many people report their depression entirely resolved by supplementing with Inositol - another B vitamin.

Low Adrenals.

In the go-go modern world where people are stretched to capacity and beyond, adrenal glands get overworked constantly. Like anything else, they can only take so much, and then they start to give out. The result is low energy, low motivation and, guess what - depression!

Various stress-reduction and stress-management techniques in combination with direct support of adrenal glands with herbs often reverse this. Two of the herbs adrenal glands 'like' the most are Ashwaganda and Licorice. (However, don't take Licorice long term if you have high blood pressure.)

Infectious Agents.

A great variety of infectious agents exist in the world, Among the most common forms are bacteria, viruses, yeast, molds, worms, parasites and spirochetes.

We all know what it feels like to be under the effect of these in acute situations like getting the flu for example - a depressing enough circumstance. But we can also be affected by chronic, low-grade infections our bodies continue to fight without our ever realizing it. These wear us down, use up our resources, make us chronically tired, vulnerable to other bugs besides the ones we've been fighting.

The ways to discover their presence can be as varied as the bugs themselves, ranging from blood tests to stool samples to muscle tests. For anyone with chronic depression symptoms, thinking "chronic low-grade infection (or infections)" can be a productive route to address.

Anemia.

This is a condition of low red blood cells. No matter what the reason, the body cells, including the brain, don't get enough oxygen when there are too few red blood cells (RBC's) This can produce depression.

Anemia can result from loss of blood, from lack of iron in the diet, from lack of absorption of iron, from stomach ulcers, medications, colon cancer, trauma or B vitamin deficiency.

Sex Hormone Imbalances.

Whether in men or women, sex hormones that are out of balance are major contributors to symptoms of depression. Therefore it's always worth it to get the levels of estrogen, progesterone and testosterone (for both men and women) checked. If any are too high or too low, they can cause depression.

Food Intolerances.

Time and time again, I've seen this as a top physical cause of depression in my clients. And the biggest food intolerance of them all is wheat, followed only by lactose and then gluten. In fact, various experts estimate that 30-50% of people are gluten intolerant, while the

WHAT IS DEPRESSION?

Depression is a common and debilitating mood disorder. More than just sadness in response to life's struggles and setbacks, depression changes how you think, feel, and function in daily activities. It can interfere with your ability to work, study, eat, sleep, and enjoy life. The feelings of helplessness, hopelessness, and worthlessness can be intense and unrelenting, with little, if any, relief.

While some people describe depression as "living in a black hole" or having a feeling of impending doom, others feel lifeless, empty, and apathetic. Men in particular can feel angry and restless. No matter how you experience depression, left untreated it can become a serious health condition. But it's important to remember that feelings of helplessness and hopelessness are symptoms of depression—not the reality of your situation. There are plenty of powerful self-help steps you can take to lift your mood, overcome depression, and regain your joy of life.

TYPES OF DEPRESSION

Here are different type of depressions

Manic Depression

Manic depression is more commonly known as Bipolar Disorder. In the case of bipolar disorder, a person experiences extreme mood swings, ranging from unbelievable highs to depressive lows. The person cannot control his/her behaviour and may take drastic steps.

Manic depression is one of the most serious forms of depression.

Persistent Depressive Disorder

If a person has undergone depression for over a period of 2 years, it is called persistent depressive disorder. Although the cause of depression may be same as major depression, for some reason the person may be incapable of overcoming it. Previously PDD was known as dysthymia.

Psychotic Depression

People suffering from psychotic depression, have symptoms similar to depression along with psychotic symptoms like hallucinations, delusions, paranoia, etc.

Seasonal Affective Disorder

It is a form of depression which is seasonal in nature, mostly happens during the winters. People who have seasonal depression, find it difficult to cope in the lack of bright sunlight. Hence during winter, their depression peaks.

Major Depression

This is the most commonly known type of depression. It is also referred to as Major Depressive Disorder. It can be caused due to any major event or even a series of smaller events or problems. A person is diagnosed with major depression if he/she displays symptoms of depression (given below types) for over two weeks.

Post-Partum Depression

This is the form of depression that women experience in the period immediately after childbirth. This could happen because of the obviously overwhelming experience, excess attention to the new born, etc.

CAUSES

It's not known exactly what causes depression. As with many mental disorders, a variety of factors may be involved, such as:

Biological differences

incidence of lactose intolerance varies by race from about 5% of the population in far Northern Europeans to 95% in native African ones.

The solution is to omit these from the diet and allow the body to detox what remains - a process that takes some time. Various authors have noted that the symptoms of manic depression (bipolar disorder) and the symptoms of gluten intolerance are exactly the same, making this a crucial factor to check when depression symptoms occur.

B Vitamin Deficiency.

There are many B vitamins we need for proper brain and nervous system functioning. Some of the more prominent ones in this regard include vitamin B1, B2, B3, B4, B5, B6 and especially B 12 and folate. Since we don't manufacture them, we require daily dietary intake to maintain healthy levels and stay out of depression.

And we also need to diminish or entirely avoid substances that strip our bodies of these essential nutrients, including refined sugars, alcohol, caffeine, and nicotine.

In many instances, what has appeared to be intractable depression is completely turned around by adequate intake of natural sources of vitamin B such as those in nutritional yeast, for example.

But don't take synthetic B vitamins - these damage the peripheral nerve plates - those tiny little nerves at the far edges of our bodies that feedback information about what's going on there to our brains so they can make adjustments.

Poor Blood Circulation.

Blockages, weaknesses or cramping in arteries negatively affect blood circulation and can result in depression for the same reason anemia does - not enough oxygen to the brain.

Where blockages exist, they can often be cleared by taking a proteolytic enzyme such as bromelain (from pineapples) on an empty stomach.

Blood vessel weaknesses are often strengthened by bioflavonoids. A rich food source of some kinds is found in the white membrane inside citrus peels, while the blue and purple range of fruits - blueberries, raspberries, grapes, bilberries - provides others.

Prescription Drugs.

Last, these are becoming a greater and greater contributor to the incidence of depression, even as more and more drugs are created to treat depression.

Therefore a careful review of any and all prescription drugs is called for when anyone suffers from depression.

And that review should include not just the drug, but all ingredients the product contains, including fillers and excipients. Two of the most common ones found in modern drugs - especially generic ones - are wheat and lactose... and these are two of the major contributors to food intolerance-generated depression.

DEPRESSION TREATMENT OPTIONS

Depression is a very life-threatening mental disorder. The suicide rates are getting higher and higher because of depression. Something needs to be done before this mental disorder turns severe. There are so many ways you can get treated from depression. Each method of treatment is different from one to another. Treatment of depression may be costly to very cheap or does not have any cost associated with it.

Treatment options that are very effective to get hold of depression are Medication, Psychotherapy, combination of Medication and Psychotherapy, Electroconvulsive therapy, self help and seeking help from others. Medication method is a bit costly method and involves side effects. Psychotherapy is a very effective option and is also a costly treatment. Other treatment methods like Self help for depression and seeking help from other people family or friends is a cost free treatment methods.

Medication

Medication is the most commonly used treatment for depression. Medicines prescribed by specialist doctors are used to cure depression. Medication treatment involves side effects. Side effects of medicines vary medicine to medicines. It is a bit expensive treatment so before going for this treatment, it is necessary to consider your pocket.

Psychotherapy

Psychotherapy is also a very effective treatment for depression. It does not involve any side effects whatsoever. Psychotherapy also referred to as "Talking therapy" Involves a depressed person and a specialist. Behavior, emotions and other things of a depressed person are focused under this treatment option. This treatment option may involves family and friends of depressed person as well as a part of whole psychotherapy process. Psychotherapy is considered as one of the premier Depression treatments. The cost of this treatment varies depending upon the accuracy of the specialist.

Electroconvulsive Therapy

Electroconvulsive therapy (ECT) is also one of the effective treatments of depression. Electric current is used in this treatment to cure depression. ECT is the fastest way to get rid of depression among all the other treatment methods. It is most effective for those that have severe depression or suicidal tendencies because of depression. It is effective in those vases as well where patient does not respond to other treatment methods. ECT may become dangerous treatment if not administrated carefully. ECT is prescribed after the treatment methods of Medication and psychotherapy under Psychiatrist's care and administration.

Apart from above most commonly used treatment methods, there are some other treatment methods for depression that help you big time. These treatment methods fall under the category of Experimental therapies. Here are some of the experimental therapies that are used by doctors on irregular basis:

- Transcranial magnetic stimulation (TMS)

- Vagal nerve stimulation (VMS)

- Hormone replacement method (HRM) especially for women.

You can also rely on other methods like self help, friends help, etc for depression treatment. Self help is the biggest treatment for depression. As the main cause of depression is our own mind. if we can do certain arrangements to get rid of those negative thoughts that lead to depression then we can easily get hold of depression to become severe from initial state.

DEPRESSION TIPS TO HANDLE THE CONDITION

There's thousands of women around the world that go through the baby blues; in fact, an amazing 80 percent are said to go through it due to the sudden drop in hormones after the birth of a baby. Most of the time, these blues disappear on their own after a couple of weeks but there are times that they can continue and turn into postpartum depression. There are some ways to handle this, whether you are looking for yourself or you are looking for a way to help your partner or friend. These postpartum depression tips are a great form of natural cures.

Exercise

This is one of the great postpartum tips as long as you have time. The good news is that you can do a dance workout in the home or buy a yoga DVD to do while the baby is asleep. Exercise releases a number of chemicals in the body, which help with the happy feelings. The exercise also helps to relax the body. All you (or your partner) need to do is 30 minutes, four days a week and you (or your partner) will be on the way to recovery.

Get Help

Sometimes, no matter how supporting friends are, the new moms will not want to talk to them. At times like this, professional help is needed. There are different types of techniques that can be used and Emotional Freedom Technique is one of them. This is through the use of pressure on the acupuncture points in the body, which will work together with the negative thoughts and fears.

Get Rest!

This is very important. The negative feelings will come out more when tiredness kicks in. The problem for new moms is that they tend to run around for everyone, whether it's the baby, the husband or even just friends. After a while, that will catch up and there is hardly any time to get some sleep. Never be afraid to ask friends for help and friends, never be afraid to offer some help around the house.

Eat Well

The body will need fuel to be able to get through the day and it's important that it is fed the right type of fuel. A healthy balanced diet is one of the best ways to get the energy that is needed. Protein and fiber are the two best options because they will release the energy slowly, which means there is more to use throughout the day.

Listen to other people's problems and try to help them

This perhaps is one of the most effective tips to get out of a brief depression (and even is useful with stress.) The mental state of depression is generated because we feel that something is wrong with oneself. So the better way to stop focusing on you is to start focusing on another person. Call a friend or family member you think may need assistance from you, provide them support unselfishly. Focusing on someone else besides your own problems may be good for you and them, the other person will be glad that you've helped in some way. Two birds with one stone.

CONCLUSION

Depression is a serious mental state, but also a temporal one. Now you have at your fingertips different ways to start dealing with this dis-ease immediately. Choose any of them and act now.

Finally, remember that if you have deep depression its always a good choice to see a psychologist. Contrary to popular opinion, the mission of the psychologist isn't "to tell you what to do" but simply to serve as a guide in order to find the solution for your problem. The truth is that sometimes another person can realize some obvious things that you on your own can't.

I LOVE YOU

I BELIVE IN YOU

YOU HAVE THE POWER!